The Cosmetic Chemicals Guide

What you need to know about the ingredients in your cosmetics and personal care products!

THE COSMETIC CHEMICALS GUIDE

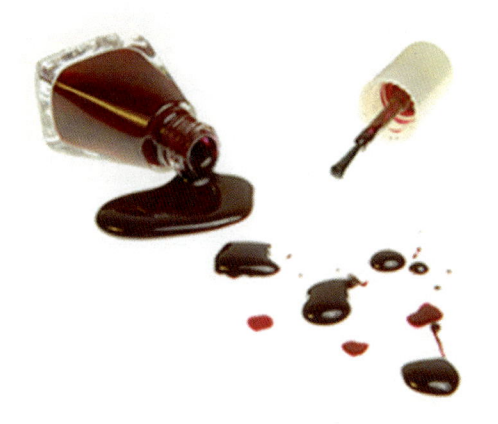

TAMARA LASCHINSKY

The Cosmetic Chemicals Guide

A look at the most common chemicals you'll find in your cosmetics and personal care products; What you should know about them before you buy!

The Cosmetic Chemicals Guide:
What You Need to Know Before You Buy
Tamara Laschinsky

First edition Copyright © 2010 Tamara Laschinsky
All rights reserved.

ISBN-13: 978-1456519018
ISBN-10: 1456519018

No part of this book may be reproduced without the written consent of the author.

Nail polish photo by: Luc Viatour   *www.Lucnix.be*

DISCLAIMER
The author has made every effort to ensure the accuracy and completeness of information in this book. Neither the author, nor publisher, assumes any responsibility for errors, inaccuracies, omissions, or any inconsistency herein.
   None of the advice found in this book should be mistaken for medical advice. Any medical concerns should be directed to a healthcare professional.

Thank you to my husband Marcus, for his love and support. This book, and my store, would not be possible without you. Thank you to my wonderful children, my initial reasons for wanting to find safer and healthier products. Thank you to my customers, for your great feedback and questions; you helped push me to find the answers.

This book is dedicated to my mother, who encouraged and inspired her children to place no limits on what could be accomplished. Every journey begins with an idea and then taking that first step forward. Thank you to my father; you made this vision become a reality and your encouragement kept me going when things got hard.

Perhaps one day, there will be a world without chemicals; a world without needless suffering and illness for our children and their children.

Thank you and love to all.

The Cosmetic Chemicals Guide

Table of Contents

～	From the Author	6
～	Why You Should Read This Book	8
～	Toxins Teen Girls Are Exposed To	9
～	Toxins Found in Umbilical Cord Blood	10
～	Chemicals @ a Glance	11
～	The FDA's Role in Assuring Safety	13
～	Toxins that "slipped in" there	14
～	Sunscreen Information	16
～	Hidden Warnings	17
～	Sneaky Marketing	18
～	Common Chemicals in Everyday Products	19
	• 1,4 Dioxane	20
	• BHA & BHT	26
	• Coal Tar	30
	• DEA, MEA & TEA	34
	• Dibutyl Phthalates	38
	• Formaldehyde Releasers	42
	• Fragrance	48
	• Methylisothiazolinone	54
	• Parabens	58
	• PEG Compounds	64
	• Petrolatum	68
	• Siloxanes	72

- Sodium Lauryl Sulfate (SLS)   76
- Triclosan   80

~ Finding More Information   84
- Online Stores   84
- EWG's Cosmetics Database   84
- David Suzuki   85
- Campaign for Safe Cosmetics   85

~ Conclusion   86

~ Resources   87

From the Author

If you had told me a few years ago that I would be an author of a book and owner of a store, I would have been quite doubtful. I had never dreamed of owning a store, and while I do enjoy writing, I had never aspired to be a published author.

Early in 2009, I encountered some extreme life-altering events. These events started a chain-reaction of experiences, which, after almost two years, has taken me up to this point.

I had seen enough illness and suffering to last a lifetime and decided that there must be something we can do about it. I felt certain the rise in health conditions such as cancer, ADHD and immune system disorders, must be somehow related to external factors and if so, then there must be some way to combat those effects.

The first step for me, was looking up all of my cosmetics and personal care products on the Skin Deep cosmetic safety database. I was shocked to see just how toxic my products were; especially those that were labelled "natural" and "organic"! The discovery led me to begin researching products that were safe and chemical-free. Once I found those products, I began ordering them for my family to use. Other moms that I knew were interested in bulking our orders together, so they too could have access to safe and chemical-free products; and that is how my store, Natural e GREEN, was formed.

What started out as a small online store, aimed at serving only my local area, grew into a very large online business serving North America. As my customer base and product line grew, so did my knowledge of chemicals and government policies surrounding cosmetics and personal care products. I spent the better part of 2010 researching, learning and writing articles on alternative health and wellness topics. With so many inquiries from customers and readers, all asking the same thing, I decided to write this book, so that everyone has access to the same knowledge I do. Knowledge is power. The more you know, the easier it will be to find safe alternatives and to demand the changes necessary to protect our children, their children and the environment.

I hope you enjoy this book and can learn about the chemical ingredients to avoid when shopping for your cosmetic and personal care products.

Slowly, manufacturers are beginning to realize that consumers are starting to pay attention and that we want safe products. One day, perhaps, this book will be obsolete because all these chemicals will be a thing of the past in consumer products. If so, then I welcome the day this book ends up in the fiction section, for it will be the day our bodies will stop being polluted by chemicals that we unknowingly use on ourselves and our children.

Why You Should Read This Book

If you are like most consumers, you aren't 100% sure of the ingredients in the products you use everyday. *This is not your fault.* The manufacturers want you, the consumer, to be in the dark and to not fully understand the potential health risks involved when using these products.

Most cosmetic and personal care products contain a variety of toxic chemicals, all of which may go under different names at times. Very few human studies have been done to determine the potential health risks. Many of these ingredients though, have been banned in proactive regions such as Europe.

It is up to you, the consumer, to see your way through the marketing hype and to decipher what the ingredients really do. This will not be easy, especially since many chemicals may not even be listed on the label.

"How is this possible?" you may ask. Sometimes, chemicals are produced during the manufacturing process and are considered by-products. By-products and contaminants are not required to be on the ingredient label. Other label ingredients, such as fragrances, do not have to disclose what compounds actually exist in the fragrance formula. We'll get into this later on.

There are hundreds upon hundreds of chemicals to be aware of when buying your cosmetic and personal care products. This book will provide you with a "short and sweet" read on the most common chemicals you'll find in your cosmetic and personal care products. You'll also find out how you can learn more about harmful chemicals and how to find safer alternatives.

Toxins Teen Girls Are Exposed To

In September 2008, the Environmental Working Group published a study conducted by Rebecca Sutton Ph.D. The study focused on determining what, if any, chemicals were present in teen-age girls' bodies. The results were quite alarming.

In a study of 20 teen girls, ages 14 - 19, 16 chemicals were found in their blood and urine. The chemicals belonged to the families of phthalates, triclosan, parabens and musks. Every single girl in the study tested positive for two types of parabens: methylparaben and propylparaben. Parabens, as we will discuss later, may be linked to breast cancer and are known endocrine disruptors.

On average, teen girls used 17 different personal care products each day, while the average adult women only uses 12. At a time when the body is changing, growing and developing, teen-agers are being exposed to wide variety of damaging chemicals. Cancer and hormonal disruption are only some of the potential health risks associated with exposure to these chemicals.

Many of these chemicals have not been studied to determine their potential health risks, but consumer awareness is on the rise and hopefully, change is on the horizon.

Toxins Found in Umbilical Cord Blood

The Environmental Working Group, EWG, published a study in 2005, in which the umbilical cord blood of newborns was analyzed for toxins. In collaboration with the Commonwealth, this study focused on 10 newborns born in August and September of 2004.

Popular belief by many scientists was that the placenta shielded cord blood and the developing fetus from toxins. This study has proved otherwise. 287 chemicals were discovered in the umbilical cord blood and it was discovered they resulted from:

- Pesticides
- Consumer product ingredients
- Waste from burning coal, gasoline and garbage
- Perfluorochemicals (used in fast food packaging)
- PFOA (Teflon chemical considered a likely carcinogen)
- Flame retardants and by-products

Of the chemicals discovered in the newborns umbilical cord blood, it is known that:

- 180 cause cancer in humans or animals
- 217 are toxic to the brain and nervous system
- 208 cause birth defects and/or abnormal development

So the question is: "Why has this never been studied before?" Perhaps more importantly, " Why are these harmful chemicals allowed by the government?" These questions are being asked more often today and the government is beginning to take notice, for the most part.

Chemicals @ a Glance

There are thousands of chemicals that can be harmful to your health, below is a list of the more common chemicals found in cosmetics and personal care products.

A - Acetone, Acetaldehyde, Acrylamide/polyacrylamide Alcohol, Alkyl-phenol Ethoxylades, Aluminum, Ammonium Glycolate, Ammonium Persulfate, Aspartame

B - Benzalkonium chloride, Cetrimonium chloride, lauryl dimonium hydrolysed collagen, Benzene, Benzoic Acid, Benzoic/Benzyl/Benzene, Benzoyl Peroxide, Bisphenol A (BPA), BHA & BHT, Bronopol, Butylparaben

C - Carboxymethylcellulose, Coal Tar Dyes, Cocamidopropyl Betaine, Coumarin

D - D&C Yellow 11, DEA: Diethanolamine, Dibutyl phthalates (DBP), Dimethicone, Dioforms, Disodium EDTA, Diazolidinyl Urea, DMDM Hydantoin

E - Ethylacrylate, Elastin

F - Fluoride, Formaldehyde, Fragrances (synthetic)

G - Glycolic Acid, GMO/Genetically Modified Organisms

H - Hydroabietyl Alcohol, Hydroquinone, Hydroxymethylcellulose

I - Imidazolidinyl Urea, Isobutylparaben, Isopropanol/Isopropyl Alcohol

K - Kajoic Acid

L - Lacquer, Lanolin, Lye

M - Magnesium Stearate/Stearic Acid
MEA: Cocamide DEA, Lauramide DEA, Linoleamide DEA,

The Cosmetic Chemicals Guide

Chemicals @ a Glance

    Oleamide DEA NDEA, Methylisothiazolinone (MIT), Methyl Methacrylate, Methylparaben, Mineral Oil

N - Nitrosamines

P - Padimate-O (PABA), Paraffin, Perchlorate, PEG Stearates, PEG (Polyethylene, polyethylene glycol, polyoxyethylene, oxynol, any ethoxylated compound including SLES), PEG-12 Distearate, PEG-80 Sorbitan Laurate, PEG-14M, Petroleum / Petrolatum, Perflurooctanotane sulfonate (PFO), Phenoxyethanol, Phthalates, Polyethylene Glycol / PEG, Polypropylene, Polyscrobate-60, Polyquaternium-7, Potassium Bromate, p-Phenylenediamine (PPD), Propylene Glycol, Propylparaben

Q - Quaternium 7, 15, 31, 60 (etc.)

S - Sodium Chloride, Sodium Hydroxymethylglycinate, Sodium Lauryl Sulfate (SLS), Sodium Laureth Sulfate (SLES), Stearalkonium Chloride

T - Talc, Triethanolamine (TEA), Toluene, Triclosan

Z - Zinc Stearate

* This is not a complete list of chemicals and many of these chemicals are known by other names and may appear under those names on product ingredient labels.

The FDA's Role in Assuring Safety

Maybe this will come as a surprise, or maybe it won't:

"Cosmetic products and ingredients are not subject to FDA pre-market approval authority, with exception of color additives."

Or this:

"The FD&C Act does not subject cosmetics to FDA pre-market approval in order to be marketed legally."

So, in a nutshell, the FDA has evaluated most ingredients used in cosmetics and personal care products and it is up the manufacturer to follow the guidelines, if any exist, when using those chemical ingredients.

"...a manufacturer may use any ingredients in the formulation of a cosmetic provided that the ingredient and the finished cosmetic are safe."

It is up to the manufacturer to:

- Ensure their product is safe before marketing.
- Ensure their product is labelled are per labeling guidelines.
- Perform their own recalls voluntarily (*FDA has no authorization to issue recalls of cosmetics*.)
- Register their cosmetics establishments (FDA does not make this mandatory, it is a voluntary program.)

Toxins that "slipped in" there

With the lack of evaluation before a product hits the market, it's no surprise to learn that products are on store shelves and contain toxins that we believe to be unsafe.

Lead in Lipstick
Dr. Lawrence E. Gibson, M.D. Mayo Clinic

Dr. Gibson indicates that very small amounts of lead have been found in some brands of lipstick. The FDA has not determined these levels to be a threat but are developing a lead test for lipstick. Currently, the FDA offers no restrictions on use of lipsticks containing lead.

Toxic Trio in Nail Polishes

Most nail polishes contained three concerning chemicals: Toluene, formaldehyde and dibutyl phthalate (DBP). While these ingredients are known to have adverse health risks, they are not illegal and may be used in nail polishes. However, consumer outcry has forced the hand of many nail polish manufacturers to voluntarily remove these toxins from their nail polishes.

1,4 Dioxane and Other By Products

There are countless other ingredients that also appear in your products, but since they are by-products of the manufacturing process, they will not appear on the labels. Current regulations do not require that they be removed from the final product.

The Cosmetic Chemicals Guide

Toxins that "slipped in" there

Contaminants in Children's Bath and Personal Care Products
The Campaign for Safe Cosmetics

48 children's bath and personal care products were independently tested for 1,4 dioxane and 28 were tested for formaldehyde.

Results:

17 out of 28 products had 1,4 dioxane and formaldehyde = 61%
23 out of 28 products had formaldehyde = 82%
32 out of 48 products had 1,4 dioxane = 67%.

Lotions, wipes, bubble bath, shampoos and soaps that tested positive for one or both toxins:

American Girl, Baby Magic, Johnson & Johnson, CVS, L'Oreal Kids, Suave Kids, Aveeno Baby, Equate, Gentle Naturals, Grins and Giggles, Huggies, Mustela, Barbie Berry, Dora the Explorer, Hot Wheels, Sesame Street, Tinker Bell.

While most of the levels of 1,4 dioxane and/or formaldehyde were low, these toxins can accumulate in the body, increasing concentration levels. Children and babies do not eliminate toxins as efficiently as adults do. A child will be exposed to these toxins from their bubble bath, from using shampoo and soap and then from using the body lotion.

1,4 dioxane is a by-product of the manufacturing process and can easily be removed by the manufacturer, though no law requires them to complete this step. Most products are put on the market with the 1,4 dioxane present in the formula.

Sunscreen Information

In the news lately is the sunscreen dilemma. Which ones work and which ones don't work? Which ones can cause hormonal disruption or poisoning?

The Environmental Working Group reported the following in their sunscreen report:

SPF = 100 (or anything 50+)
These sunscreens look promising but, while they do protect you from UVB rays and sunburns, *they provide little or no protection from UVA rays* (the ones that penetrate deep and can cause cancer.)

Mineral Powder SPF
These brush on sunscreens do contain zinc and titanium and offer strong protection, but there is little control of the particles when brushing all over your body and the particles can end up in your lungs and enter your bloodstream. Inhaled titanium dioxide may be carcinogenic, according to the International Agency for Research on Cancer.

Oxybenzone Ingredients
Great for blocking the sun's rays but is also a suspected endocrine disruptor. It is not recommended for applying over a large area of your body. Labeling guidelines say manufacturers must give the consumer fair warning and so, you will see instructions such as "apply liberally" or "use sparingly."

"Natural" Labels
Beware the word "natural" and look extra close when reading the ingredients. Some brands, labeled "natural" have many ingredients that do not occur in nature; many are made from petroleum.

Hidden Warnings

While many ingredients and chemical compounds are allowed in products (with restrictions), manufacturers may not have to disclose what they are.

If the product contains a by-product, the chemical would be considered a "contaminant" and is not required to be printed on the label.

The same is said for fragrances. Fragrances are a "trade secret" that manufacturers are allowed to keep private. Fragrances are often made up of various chemical compounds, some of which are known to be harmful to your health.

Manufacturers must put warnings on their products if it is known to contain an ingredient that may have serious health risks. Look for the following terms:

> " Keep out of reach of children."
> " Keep away from children."
> " Use under adult supervision."
> " If ingested, contact your local Poison Control Centre."
> " Keep away from eyes."
> " Discontinue use if rash occurs; consult doctor if symptoms worsen or persist."

Those warnings labels are not put there because the manufacturers care, they are there because labeling regulations require them to be there. Those warnings mean that the product contains one or more ingredients that are known to be harmful to human health. *Watch for the warnings!*

Sneaky Marketing

Have you ever taken a marketing course? I actually majored in it and understand it all too well. Marketing is all about: *"Perception."* How a consumer perceives an idea or product and making sure the perception results in an action (such as buying the product.)

I'm a victim too. I am a sucker for marketing ploys that design products to look natural & healthy (perception of course!).

Watch for this:

- Packaging that has "earth tones" (greens, beiges, browns, blues)
- Images of trees, leaves, grasses, flowers
- The famous words "natural", "herbal" or "pure". Be cautious of the word "organic" because even a product with one or two "organic" ingredients can still be mixed in with the not-so-good chemicals!

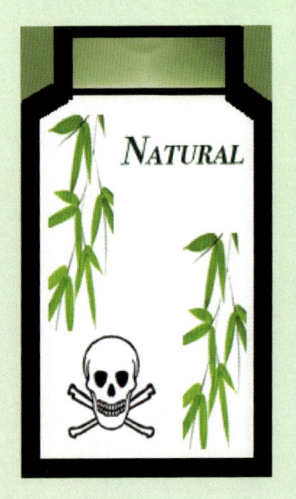

When you see these products that make you think "*safe*", "*healthy*", "*pure*", "*gentle*", "*good for you*" and "*nature*", take a read on the ingredients list. If you're not sure what they all mean, look them up on the EWG's cosmetic database and get the real truth!

Fact: Chemicals are cheap and allow mass production of low cost goods for lower prices. Most store brands contain some nasty chemicals in them. It does not matter what their packaging looks like, who's endorsing it or how popular they are. Read the ingredients; knowledge is power!

The Cosmetic Chemicals Guide

Common Chemicals in Everyday Products

If you've been to the store lately and picked up a personal care product, you may have been interested in reading the ingredients label on the back. Reading the label is one thing; understanding it is another!

Many ingredients have ridiculously long names, and it makes it hard to understand what they are. Adding to the confusion is the recent introduction of many essential oils and natural ingredients, as their descriptive names are often quite lengthy and can be mistaken for synthetic chemical names.

So how do you decipher the ingredient listings and feel good (and safe) about what you are using? It won't be easy. Having a basic understanding to the common chemicals to watch for when reading labels is the first step. While many chemical compounds have alternate names they may go under, you can often pick them up by their prefixes or other designations.

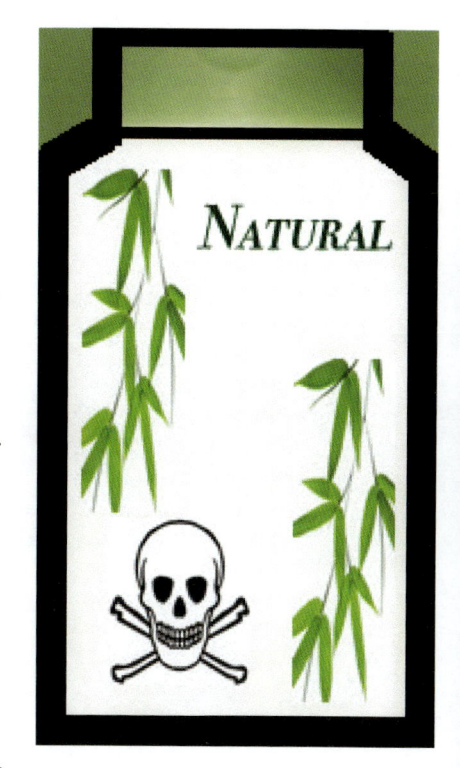

Doing your research and comparing your products to resource sites such as the Environmental Working Group's "Cosmetic Database", will also aid you in your quest for safer products.

19

The Cosmetic Chemicals Guide

1,4 Dioxane

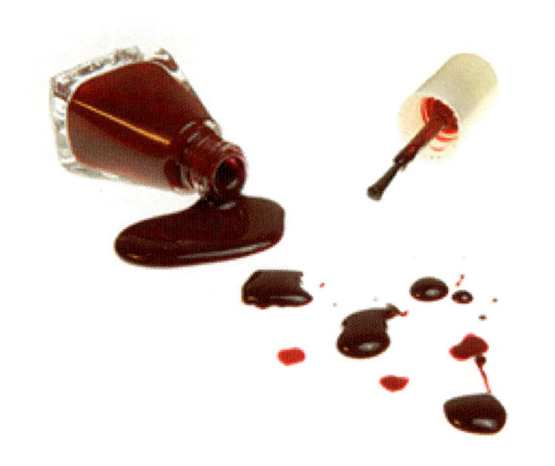

The Cosmetic Chemicals Guide

1,4 Dioxane

Used As: Unwanted by-product, carcinogen. According to EWG, contaminates up to 46% of personal care products. Banned/unsafe for use in cosmetics. (May not be deliberately added to product but can appear as a by-product)

Dangers:
- ➡ Skin, eye and lungs irritant
- ➡ Human immune system toxicant
- ➡ Reproductive effects
- ➡ Respiratory toxicant
- ➡ Cancer - strong evidence

Found In:
- ☑ Body washes and soaps
- ☑ Detergents
- ☑ Toothpastes
- ☑ Shampoo, conditioners
- ☑ Muscle rubs
- ☑ Hair styling
- ☑ Body oils
- ☑ Cosmetics

Also known as:

1,4 -Diethylene Dioxide, 1,4 - Dioxacyclohexane, Di(Ethylene Oxide), Diethylene Dioxide, Diethylene Dioxide (Osha), Diethylene Ether, Diokan, Dioksan (Polish) Diossanoa - 1,4 (Italian), Dioxaan-1,4 (Dutch), Dioxan

Did You Know? *1,4 Dioxane is known to cause cancer and while manufacturers could easily remove it from the product, most often they do not.*

1,4 Dioxane

Hazards

Cancer concerns	Strong evidence indicates that 1,4 Dioxane is a human carcinogen. Banned by the European Union (EU), flagged by the Canadian Environmental Protection Act (CEPA).
Irritant	Classified as irritant to skin, eyes or lungs. Prolonged exposure may lead to dermatitis.
Reproductive effects	Animal studies show reproductive effects.
Identifying challenges	By-products are not required to be on ingredient label. Cautionary statements such as " *keep out of reach of children*", or, "*use under adult supervision*", may indicate potential 1,4 Dioxane by-product.

Environment Canada Domestic Substances List: *Classified as suspected to be carcinogenic*

1,4 Dioxane

So what have you learned about 1,4 Dioxane?

→ 1,4 Dioxane is a by-product of the manufacturing process. While it could easily be removed by the manufacturer, by a process known as vacuum stripping, most times it is not.

→ Since by-products are not required by law to be listed on the ingredients label, you have no definite way of knowing whether or not you're being exposed to 1,4 Dioxane. Your best line of defense is avoiding the known chemicals that can produce 1,4 Dioxane.

→ The European Union has banned 1,4 Dioxane from it's products and the Canadian Environmental Protection Act has flagged 1,4 Dioxane for further investigation.

→ 1,4 Dioxane can also cause allergic reactions on the skin and in the lungs.

→ The U.S. Food & Drug Administration, FDA, indicates products that may contain the impurity may include the prefix of designations or *"PEG,"* *"-eth"*, *"Polyethylene"*, *"Polyethylene glycol"*, *"Polyoxyethylene"*, or *"-oxynol-"*.

In the News

Procter & Gamble (P&G) announced during a press conference that it would reformulate 18 different Herbal Essences products in order to reduce the toxic chemical: 1,4 dioxane. This action was prompted so that P&G would be in accordance with California's Proposition 65, which states that 1,4 dioxane can not exceed more than 10 parts per million (ppm) in consumer products.

The Green Patriot Working Group (GPWG) along with the Organic Consumers Association (OCA) and the Campaign for Safe Cosmetics and Clean Water Action California, were able to sway P&G to making the right decision regarding reformulating the products.

1,4 Dioxane is a by-product of the manufacturing process and if it is not directly added to the product, it is not required to appear on the ingredient label. However, just because it has not been directly added to the product does not mean it is not present. Manufacturers can remove the product before putting it on the market, but most do not do this final step.

As Canwest News Service reported in September of 2009, a recommendation was put forth to designate 1,4 Dioxane as "toxic" under the Canadian Environmental Protection Act. Unfortunately, the recommendation was denied and Health Canada decided that this possibly carcinogenic chemical will not be added to that list. The chemical is often found in trace amounts in product such as baby shampoo, bubble bath and soaps.

The thought behind the ruling is that the trace amounts of the chemical do not expose the consumer to the doses of 1,4 Dioxane that are known to be a health risk. However, with 1,4 Dioxane present is so many cosmetics and personal care products, it is uncertain what levels consumers are exposed to on a daily basis and just how much accumulates in your body.

While the U.S Food and Drug Administration "recommends" that cosmetic products should not contain 1,4 Dioxane in concentrations greater than 10 ppm, many products exceed that amount and use of various products would expose consumers to levels higher than FDA recommendations.

The Alliance for A Healthier Tomorrow displayed the 2007 results of over two dozen products that were independently tested by West Coast Analytical Service. Found to be just at, or over, the FDA recommendations were:

- Hello Kitty Bubble Bath   12 ppm
- Johnson's Kids Shampoo Watermelon Explosion   10 ppm
- Clairol Herbal Essences Rainforest Flowers Shampoo   23 ppm
- Olay Complete Body Wash with Vitamins   23 ppm

With no pre-market testing required by the FDA, many products can contain these chemicals and exceed FDA recommendations.

The Cosmetic Chemicals Guide

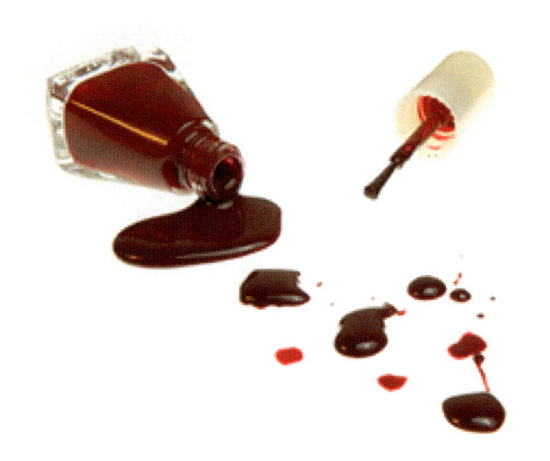

BHA & BHT

The Cosmetic Chemicals Guide

BHA & BHT

Used As: Used as preservatives in cosmetics and also as food preservative. Also used as a fragrance.

Dangers:
➡ Skin and eye irritant
➡ Immune system toxicant
➡ Reproductive effects
➡ Endocrine disruption
➡ Toxic to organs
➡ Mammalian cells showed positive mutation results

Found In:
☑ Body washes and soaps
☑ Lubricants and body oils
☑ Cosmetics
☑ Nail polish removers
☑ Deodorants
☑ Food
☑ Sunscreens

Did You Know? BHA has been classified by the U.S National Toxicology Program as "reasonably anticipated to be a human carcinogen" based on animal studies.

Also known as:

Antioxyne B,

Antrancine 12,

EEC No. E320,

Embanox,

Nipantiox 1-F,

Protex, Sustane 1-F, Tenox BHA,

DBPC, Advastab 401, Agidol, Agidol 1, Alkofen BP,

Antioxidant (29) (30) (4K) (K8),

Antrancine 8.

27

The Cosmetic Chemicals Guide

BHA & BHT

Hazards

Endocrine disruption	Has shown to be an endocrine disruptor in animal studies. Strong evidence it's a human endocrine disruptor.
Environmental concerns	Persistent and bioaccumulative in wildlife. Harmful to environment and chemical of concern.
Irritant	Can induce allergic reactions.
Cancer concerns	Suspected of being a human carcinogen. Flagged by the CEPA for carcinogenic concerns.
Restrictions	Banned by the European Union; found to be unsafe in cosmetics.

Environment Canada Domestic Substances List:	*Classified as suspected to have carcinogenic properties.*

BHA & BHT

So what have you learned about BHA & BHT?

➡ BHA and BHT are synthetic antioxidants and are closely related. Both are used as preservatives for cosmetics and foods.

➡ BHA and BHT can both induce allergic skin reactions.

➡ Possible carcinogen and deemed a "high human health priority" by Health Canada. Also flagged for further investigation.

➡ Long term exposure of BHT in mice and rats has shown to be toxic. It may also mimic estrogen and lead to reproductive effects for both females and males.

➡ BHA is banned by the European Union as a fragrance ingredient in cosmetics.

➡ State of California requires products containing BHA to have warning labels.

The Cosmetic Chemicals Guide

Coal Tar

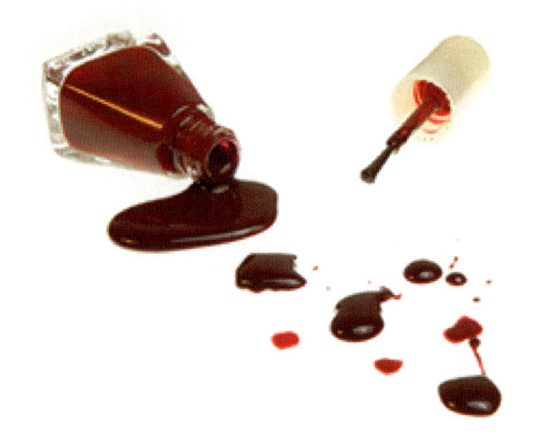

The Cosmetic Chemicals Guide

Coal Tar Dyes

Used As: Antidandruff agent. Biocide to prevent growth of organisms. Color.

Dangers:
➡ Skin and eye irritant
➡ Reproductive effects
➡ Respiratory toxicant
➡ Persistence and bioaccumulation
➡ Environmental toxin
➡ Known carcinogen

Found In:
☑ Hair dyes (the darker the dye the more p-phenylenediamine is found)
☑ Antidandruff shampoos
☑ Skin disorder treatments
☑ Some lipsticks & cosmetics

Did You Know? **FD&C** *means approved for use in* **F**ood, **D**rugs and **C**osmetics. **D&C** *means only approved for use in* **D**rugs & **C**osmetics. *Coal tar colors can be D&C, therefore, not approved for ingestion, but can be allowed for lipsticks which may be accidentally ingested.*

Also known as:

P-phenylenediamine, CI (followed by 5 digit #'s) Tar, Coal, Coal Tar Solution, Carbo-Cort, Coal Tar Solution US, Coal Tar Aerosol, Crude Coal Tar, Estar (Skin Treatment), Impervotar KC 261, Lavatar, PICIS Carbonis

Coal Tar Dyes

Hazards

Cancer concerns	Recognized as a human carcinogen. *P-phenylenediamine* has been found to cause cancer in studies done by the U.S. National Cancer Institute and the National Toxicology Program.
Immune system sensitizer	Can produce immune system responses such as itching, scaling, hives, burning and blistering of skin.
Restrictions	Banned or restricted in cosmetics in the European Union. Also prohibited and restricted for use in Canadian cosmetics.
Environmental concerns	Toxic when it comes in contact with aquatic organisms and is persistent and bioaccumulative.

Environment Canada Domestic Substances List:	*Classified as suspected to be persistent, carcinogenic and toxic to aquatic life.*

The Cosmetic Chemicals Guide

Coal Tar Dyes

So what have you learned about Coal Tar Dyes?

➡ Coal Tar is a mix of many different types of chemicals and is derived from petroleum.

➡ Coal Tar-derived colors are used is cosmetics and will often show as a 5-digit Index (CI) number. "FD&C Blue No. 1" or "Blue 1" are some examples or coal-tar derived color.

➡ Coal Tar-derived colors may be deemed unsafe for use in food products but allowed in cosmetics such as lipstick, that may be accidentally ingested.

➡ Hair dyes often contain p-phenylenediamine. Darker colors contain more p-phenylenediamine.

➡ P-phenylenediamine has proved to be carcinogenic in laboratory tests conducted by the U.S National Cancer Institute and the National Toxicology Program.

➡ Coal Tar ingredients are used in some antidandruff products.

➡ Coal Tar ingredients are used in creams and lotions used to treat severe dermatitis, eczema and psoriasis.

➡ P-phenylenediamine is only allowed in hair dyes and product labels must carry the warning " contains ingredients that may cause skin irritation and certain individuals" and if product is to be used near the eyes, " may cause blindness."

The Cosmetic Chemicals Guide

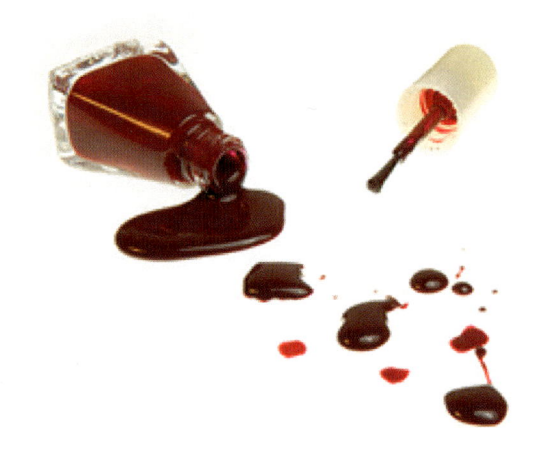

DEA, MEA & TEA

34

The Cosmetic Chemicals Guide

DEA, MEA, TEA

Used As: As a pH adjuster. Makes cosmetics creamy or sudsy.

Dangers:
- Skin, eye and lung irritant
- Neurotoxicity
- Reproductive effects
- Cardiovascular effects
- Endocrine disruption
- Toxicity to aquatic organisms.
- May form nitrosamines (can cause cancer)

Found In:
- ☑ Sunblock
- ☑ Facial cleansers
- ☑ Anti-itch creams
- ☑ Tinted moisturizers
- ☑ Soaps & washes
- ☑ Shampoos

Also known as:

Diethanolamine, N,N-Diethanolamine, 2,2'-Dihydroxydiethylamine, 2,2'-Iminobisethanol, 2,2'-Iminodiethanol, 2-Hydroxethylamino, Cocomide DEA, Amides, Coco, Coco Fatty Acid Amide, Coco Amides, Coconut Diethanolamide, Cocoyl Diethanolamide

Did You Know? MEA and TEA are related chemicals to DEA and can react with other chemicals to form carcinogenic nitrosamines.

The Cosmetic Chemicals Guide

DEA, MEA, TEA

Hazards

Irritant	Irritant to skin, eyes and lungs. Harmful if swallowed.
Immune system response	Can trigger skin reaction of blistering, hives, scaling, itching and burning sensation.
Air pollutant	Clean Air Act deems DEA to be a hazardous air pollutant.
Cancer concerns	Can react with nitrates to form nitrosamines. Nitrosamines are linked to various types of cancer. Nitrates are added as anti-corrosive agents or be present as contaminants or by-products.

Environment Canada Domestic Substances List: *Considered a moderate human health priority and flagged for further review.*

The Cosmetic Chemicals Guide

DEA, MEA & TEA

So what have you learned about DEA, MEA & TEA?

➡ Diethanolamine, is also known as DEA, Cocomide DEA and Lauramide DEA

➡ Related chemicals to DEA are MEA (monoethanolamide) and TEA (triethanolamine).

➡ DEA, MEA, TEA have the ability to react with nitrates and form nitrosamines which are suspected of causing various types of cancer.

➡ Deemed hazardous to the environment by The Danish Environmental Protection Agency due to toxicity to aquatic organisms.

➡ Hazardous air pollutant and can cause respiratory illness.

➡ Cocomide DEA is coconut oil that has been chemically-modified to act as a foaming agent.

➡ Found in many soaps, cleansers and shampoos.

The Cosmetic Chemicals Guide

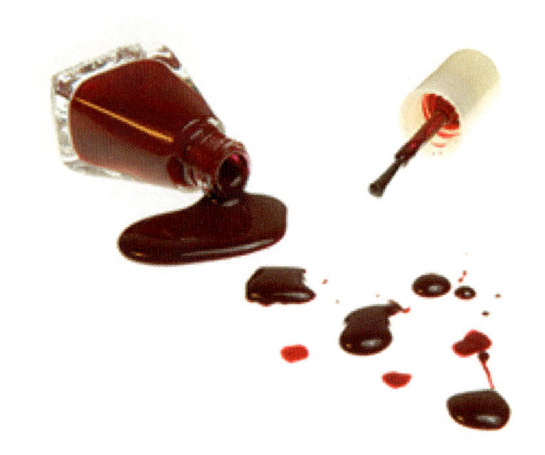

Dibutyl Phthalates

The Cosmetic Chemicals Guide

Dibutyl Phthalates

Used As: Solvent for dyes in nail products and as plasticizer to keeps nail polishes from becoming brittle. Fragrance ingredient.

Dangers:
- Allergies and skin sensitivities
- Neurotoxicity
- Endocrine disruption
- Environmental toxin
- Biochemical changes (animal studies)
- Reproductive and development toxin

Found In:
- ☑ Nail polishes
- ☑ Nail treatments

Did You Know? Health Canada recently banned use of six phthalates (including DBP) in children's toys and articles, but has not banned its use in cosmetic products!

Also known as:

1,2-Benzenedicarboxylic Acid, Dibutyl Ester, Dibutyl 1,2-Benzenedicarboxylate, DBP, Dibutyl Phthalate, DI-N-Butylphthalate, Benzene-O-Dicarboxylic Acid, Di-N_Butyl Ester, Celluflex DPB, Di-N-Butyl Phthalate

The Cosmetic Chemicals Guide

Dibutyl Phthalates

Hazards

Reproductive organs and endocrine disruption	May be toxic to the reproductive system, possible cause harm to unborn baby. Risk of impaired fertility. Endocrine disruptor. The state of California has classified DBP as a reproductive and developmental toxicant.
Fragrances	Reported to be used in fragrance ingredients; fragrance labels do not have to include chemicals used in making the fragrance.
Restrictions	Banned by the European Union for use in cosmetics and personal care products.
Environmental concerns	Clean Air Act deems DBP a water pollutant. Suspected to be toxic to aquatic life. Persistent and bioaccumulative.
Irritant	Can cause allergic reactions.

Environment Canada Domestic Substances List: *Classified as expected to be toxic or harmful.*

40

Dibutyl Phthalates

So what have you learned about Phthalates?

➡ Used in nail polishes, lacquers and treatments as solvent and to keep product from becoming brittle.

➡ Banned by Health Canada in children's toys and articles, but not in cosmetics.

➡ Banned by the European Union for use in cosmetics and personal care products.

➡ Suspected of being harmful to reproductive system and of causing harm to the unborn child.

➡ Dangerous to the environment and aquatic life.

➡ Used in fragrances but due to fragrance privacy rights, does not need to be included on the label when used as part of the fragrance formula. If product indicates "fragrance" or "parfum" on their ingredients label, there is the possibility that DBP is present.

➡ Can be irritating and cause skin allergic reactions.

The Cosmetic Chemicals Guide

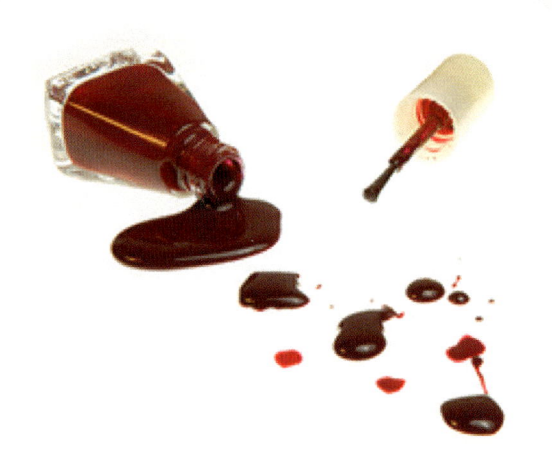

Formaldehyde Releasers

The Cosmetic Chemicals Guide

Formaldehyde Releasers

Used As: Preservative. Biocide to prevent growth of organisms.

Dangers:
➡ Cancer causing ingredient
➡ Immune system toxicant
➡ Cause skin irritation and burns
➡ Respiratory toxicant
➡ Cardiovascular toxicant
➡ Neurotoxicity
➡ Environmental toxin

Found In:
☑ Baby bath products
☑ Adult bath products
☑ Hair care
☑ Cosmetics
☑ Diaper wipes
☑ Lotions
☑ Sunscreens

Also known as:

Formalin, Formic Aldehyde, Merthaldehyde, Methanal, Methyl Aldehyde, Oxomethane, Oxymethylene, Aldehyde Mravenci (Czech), Aldehyde Formique (French), Aldeide Formica (Italian) BFV, DMDM hydantoin, diazolidinyl urea, imidazolidinyl urea, methenamine, quaternium-15, sodium hydroxymethylglycinate, 1,3-Bis (Hydroxymethyl), 1,3 Dimethylol, 5,5-Dimethylhydantoin, Chloroallyl Methenamine Chloride, 2,5-Dioxo-4-Imidazolidinyl

Did You Know? Formaldehyde by itself is restricted to not exceed concentrations of 0.2 percent in most products, but there are no restrictions placed on other chemical ingredients that release formaldehyde in low-levels.

The Cosmetic Chemicals Guide

Formaldehyde Releasers

Hazards

Cancer	Known human carcinogen.
Irritant	Cause irritation to skin, eyes and lungs. Corrosive and can cause burns.
Reproductive	Has an effect on the menstrual cycle, may be toxic to the reproductive system.
Further studies	While formaldehyde itself is not flagged for further review (since it's health risks are already well known), other chemical that release formaldehyde, such as quaternium-15, are flagged for further review by the CEPA.
Neurotoxicity	Animal studies show brain, nervous system or behavioral effects.
Environmental	Suspected to be an environmental toxin.
Organs	Toxic to organs.

Environment Canada Domestic Substances List: *Formaldehyde releasing chemicals flagged for further review.*

44

Formaldehyde Releasers

So what have you learned about Formaldehyde Releasers?

➡ Formaldehyde is a known human carcinogen

➡ In most Canadian products, formaldehyde may not exceed 0.2 percent concentration. Nail hardeners may contain up to 5 percent concentration.

➡ Products containing more than 0.05 percent formaldehyde-releasing chemicals in the European Union, must carry the warning *"contains formaldehyde"* on their labels.

➡ Formaldehyde occurs naturally in the environment.

➡ Formaldehyde has many names and can be found as a by-product from other chemicals.

➡ Nail polishes used to contain formaldehyde but due to consumer pressure, many major cosmetic companies have voluntarily removed formaldehyde from the ingredients.

➡ There are no requirements to test products that contain formaldehyde-releasing chemicals or to determine the levels of formaldehyde they release.

In the News

October 2010 - Brazilian Blowout, a popular hair straightening formula, made headlines when dangerously high levels of formaldehyde were discovered.

The expensive treatment used by many celebrities, including Jennifer Aniston, Lindsay Lohan and Reese Witherspoon, was removed from shelves following public health warnings.

Staff at an Oregon salon complained of eye irritation, bleeding noses and breathing problems after using the formula. Chemists tested the product and found that although the product was labeled "formaldehyde-free", it contained significant levels of formaldehyde.

Manufacturers are required to notify salon workers if any product contains more than 0.1 percent formaldehyde; Brazilian Blowout contained between 4.85 percent to 10.6 percent formaldehyde.

The general public is exposed to formaldehyde through certain foods and products and The U.S Centers for Disease Control and Prevention indicates that even low exposure can cause irritation to the eyes, skin, nose and throat. High and long-term levels of exposure have been linked to human cancer.

The Occupation Health and Safety Administration reports that until salon workers can be sure a product contains no formaldehyde, they should always wear masks, goggles and respirators.

Health Canada stopped distribution of Brazilian Blowout, when their own testing of the product showed formaldehyde levels of 12%. It was believed the formaldehyde became airborne during the blow drying and flat iron stages of the treatment and at levels that high, placed both the clients and stylists at risk.

The manufacturer claimed, at first, that the product did not contain any formaldehyde, and was going to do independent reviews.

In Canada, even though salons were warned about the product's danger, some salons continued to offer the treatment to clients without acknowledging the potential health hazards. These salons were offering the treatment at discounted prices, until the manufacturer finally stopped shipments of the product.

The Cosmetic Chemicals Guide

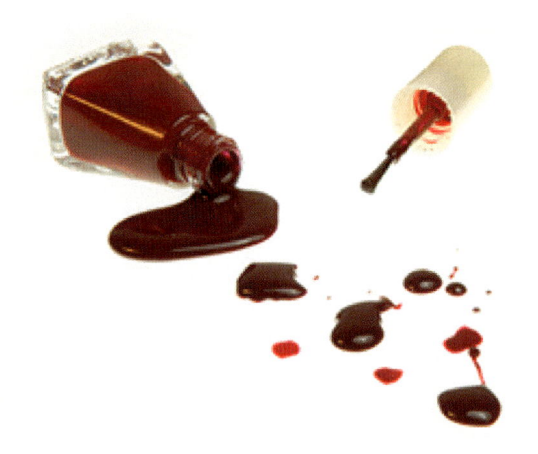

Fragrance

Fragrance

Used As: Deodorant, to mask scents and to add pleasant scents to product.

Also known as:

Parfum, Scent

Dangers:
- ➡ Allergies
- ➡ Reproductive effects
- ➡ Dermatitis
- ➡ Respiratory effects

Found In: ☑ All products
• *Shampoos, conditioners, lotions, creams, makeup, bath products, body oils, soaps, laundry detergents, deodorants, perfumes, air fresheners, diaper creams, diaper wipes, hand sanitizer, sunscreens, lip balms, cleaning products*

Did You Know? Fragrances are "trade secrets" and made up of different chemical compounds, some of which are known to cause harmful health problems. Since they are considered "trade secrets", the individual chemicals in fragrances do not need to be listed or disclosed to the consumer.

Fragrance

Hazards

Allergies & dermatitis	Ingredients in fragrances are often irritants and can irritate asthma, allergic reactions and dermatology conditions.
Hormone disruptors	Use of diethyl phthalate (DEP) to make scent linger is also known to disrupt hormonal levels and impact reproductive organs.
Environmental concerns	Synthetic musks pose environmental concerns due to their tendency to be persistent and bioaccumulative. Synthetic musks levels are rising in the Great Lakes and in the fish living in the Great Lakes.
Accumulation	A study done by the Environmental Working Group, shows that common synthetic musk was found present in umbilical cord blood of 7 out of 10 newborns.

Environment Canada Domestic Substances List: *Not flagged for further review at this time.*

Fragrance

So what have you learned about Fragrance?

➡ Fragrances are found in almost every product on store shelves, with the exception of most food products.

➡ Fragrances are chemical mixtures, composed of many different chemicals and interactions.

➡ They only need to be listed as "Fragrance" or "Parfum" as they are considered "trade secrets." Consumers do not have the right to know what specific ingredients are in a fragrance or parfum.

➡ Many harmful chemical compounds have been found in fragrances.

➡ Fragrance ingredients used for "masking" purposes are designed to prevent your brain from perceiving the fragrance scent. Products that say "fragrance-free" or "unscented" may still contain fragrance ingredients that fool your brain into believing the product contains no scent at all.

➡ Phthalates, commonly used in fragrances to make the scent linger and last longer, have been linked to hormonal disruption, reproductive damage, liver and kidney failure in young children, obesity, insulin resistance in men and are harmful to the environment.

In the News

Besides possibly containing chemicals in their "secret" formulas, fragrances are also well known to cause allergic reactions. People with chemical sensitivities are often affected by fragrances and individual reactions vary.

In December 2010, the Toronto Sun composed a news article on chemical sensitivity. Chemical sensitivity is when an individual is very sensitive to certain chemicals; especially fragrances.

For some, synthetic fragrances are more likely to bring on a reaction, while essential oils remain relatively safe. Most people with chemical sensitivities avoid wearing perfumes, but in this day and age of scents fragrance is everywhere and quite difficult to avoid.

In public, exposure to fragrance can be high and unavoidable. Other people, such as co-workers, wearing perfumes can trigger allergic reactions. Many businesses and stores use air fresheners, which can also bring on reactions.

Chemical sensitivity can be a debilitating ailment and can be very harmful to an individual's health. While even essential oils can bring on reactions, synthetic fragrances, with their list of chemical ingredients, are more likely to cause any of the following symptoms:

- Itchy eyes
- Runny nose
- Headaches and migraines
- Concentration issues and/or confusion
- Anxiety or depression
- Muscle aches

The Cosmetic Chemicals Guide

- Tingling sensation on lips or skin
- Respiratory issues (coughing, wheezing)
- Nausea or vomiting
- Increase in asthma attacks
- Skin rashes (eczema, hives)
- Anaphylactic Shock

The Canadian Human Rights Commission recognizes an individual's right to be protected from fragrances. More businesses and organizations are introducing scent-free policies which help to protect those with sensitivities.

The Cosmetic Chemicals Guide

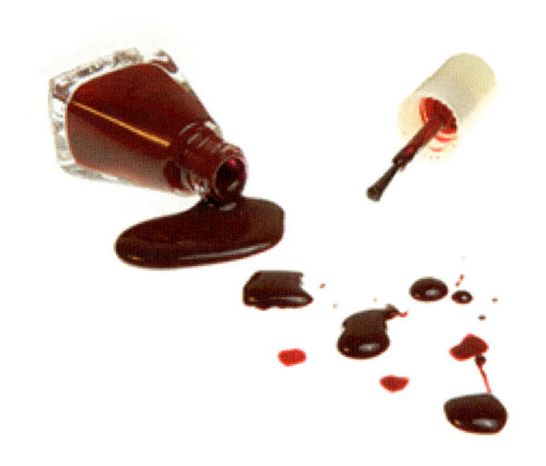

Methylisothiazolinone (MIT)

The Cosmetic Chemicals Guide

Methylisothiazolinone (MIT)

Used As: A preservative.

Dangers:
→ Immune system toxicant
→ Skin toxicant
→ Allergies
→ Neurotoxic

Found In:
- ☑ Baby sunscreen lotion
- ☑ Hand washes and sanitizer
- ☑ Lubricants
- ☑ Shaving cream
- ☑ Moisturizing lotion
- ☑ Baby wipes
- ☑ Facial cleansers
- ☑ Hair products
- ☑ Bath & shower gel and oils
- ☑ Cosmetics

Also known as:

3 (2H) - Isothiazolone, 2-Methyl-; Methylchloroisothiazolinone225Methylisothiazolinone solution; 2-Methyl-3 (2H) - Isothiazolone; 2-Methyl-4-Isothiazolin-3-one; 2-Methyl- 3 (2H) - Isothiazolone; 2-Methyl-2H-Isothiazol-3-One; 3 (2H) Isothiazolone, 2Methyl; 2-Methyl-3 (2H) - Isothiazolone; 2-Methyl-4-Isothiazolin-3-One

Did You Know? MIT is known to cause skin irritations but further studies are needed to understand other potential health risks.

The Cosmetic Chemicals Guide

Methylisothiazolinone (MIT)

Hazards

Skin allergies	MIT is known to cause skin irritation.
Neurotoxicity	Suspected to be highly toxic to neurons according to in-vitro studies.
Immune system sensitizer	Can produce itching, burning, hives, scaling and blistering of the skin as a reaction.

Environment Canada Domestic Substances List:	*Not flagged for further investigation at this time.*

Methylisothiazolinone (MIT)

So what have you learned about MIT?

➡ MIT is used as a preservative in many cosmetic, personal care and cleaning products.

➡ MIT is commonly used to replace parabens in products.

➡ It is known to cause allergic skin reactions.

➡ Use is restricted in Canadian cosmetics and must not exceed maximum concentrations.

➡ In Japan, concentration limits exist when MIT is used in combination with other ingredients.

➡ In-vitro tests showed MIT to be toxic to mammalian cells.

➡ Further testing of this ingredients must be done to assess other possible health risks.

The Cosmetic Chemicals Guide

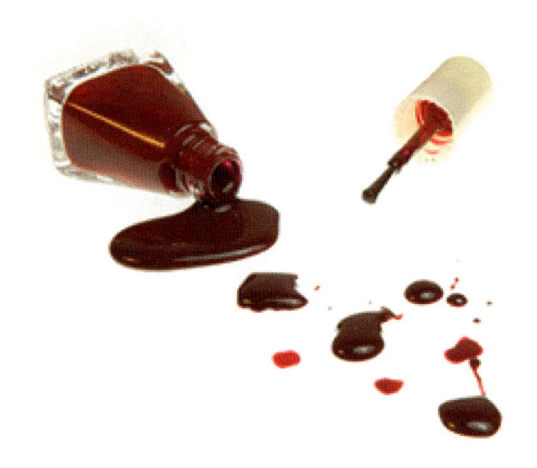

Parabens

The Cosmetic Chemicals Guide

Parabens
(methyl, ethyl, butyl, propyl, isopropyl)

Used As: Fragrance ingredient and preservative.

Dangers:
➡ Allergies (skin, eyes, lungs)
➡ Endocrine disruption
➡ Mammalian cell disruption (cancer)
➡ Neurotoxicity

Found In:
☑ Food sources
☑ Hair care products
☑ Lotions and creams
☑ Cosmetics
☑ Deodorant
☑ Sunscreen
☑ Baby lotions, creams
☑ Shower gels, bath products
☑ Lubricants

Also known as:

Benzoic Acid, 4-Hydroxy-, Methyl Ester, P-Carbomrhoxyphenol, Methylparaben, potassium salt, Propyl Ester, Propyl Ester Sodium Salt, Ethyl Ester, Ethyl 4-Hydroxybenzoate, Ethyl P-Hydroxybenzoate, 1-Methylethyl Ester, Isopropyl Ester

Did You Know? It is estimated that 75% - 90% of cosmetics contain low-levels of parabens.

Parabens
(methyl, ethyl, butyl, propyl, isopropyl)

Hazards

Skin absorption	Can easily penetrate the skin and enter the bloodstream.
Endocrine disruption	Parabens mimic estrogen, the female sex hormone. Can result in lower sperm counts for men.
UVB interaction	When methylparaben was applied to the skin, and allowed to react with UVB rays, increased skin aging and DNA damage occurred.
Cancer	Parabens have been found in breast cancer tumors and suspected to be linked to the progression of breast cancer.

Environment Canada Domestic Substances List: *Not flagged for further investigation at this time.*

The Cosmetic Chemicals Guide

Parabens

(methyl, ethyl, butyl, propyl, isopropyl)

So what have you learned about Parabens?

➡ Parabens are widely used as a preservative in personal care products and cosmetics.

➡ They are known to mimic estrogen, though full health risks are not fully understood

➡ Parabens were detected in breast tumor tissue (*Darbre, in the Journal of Applied Toxicology 2004*), though further studies must be done to determine if the parabens caused the cancer, increased cancer progression or were just coincidental.

➡ Cosmetics often have low-levels of parabens, however, with the average woman using more than 10 different personal care products each day, the total paraben exposure and accumulation is not known.

➡ There are no restrictions on the use of parabens in cosmetics, nor any regulations surrounding the use of parabens in these products.

➡ In Denmark, parabens have recently been banned for use in products used for children ages 0 - 3 years.

In the News

December 2010 - Denmark became the first European country to ban use of parabens in children's products for children under the age of three. Propylparaben and butylparaben are no longer allowed to be present in these children's products.

In 2006, the European Commission listed parabens as a Category 1 substance, which indicates it shows evidence of causing endocrine disruption.

In June 2010, the U.S. Centers for Disease Control and Prevention took notice of the chemical preservative, after a study concluded that parabens were widely present in urine samples of participants. The study collected 2,548 urine samples of adults and children ages six years and older. The results were shocking:

- 99.1% tested positive for methylparaben
- 92.7% tested positive for propylparaben
- 42.4% tested positive for ethylparaben
- 47% tested positive for butylparaben

The study also concluded that females has significantly higher concentrations of methylparaben in their bodies than males did.

Parabens were discovered by British researchers to be present in the tissue of women who suffered from breast cancer. 20 samples of human breast tissue were tested and all had traces of at least one type of paraben.

The study can not conclude that parabens are linked directly to causing cancer; it can only prove that parabens do accumulate in the body. Further testing is now underway to determine the effects of parabens on human health and the dangers they may pose.

Despite the government's indecision on the harmful effects of parabens on human health, consumers are beginning to look for paraben-free alternatives. Testing of parabens on human health may take years of studies and analysis, some manufacturers are listening to consumer requests and working on paraben-free formulas to offer customers.

The Cosmetic Chemicals Guide

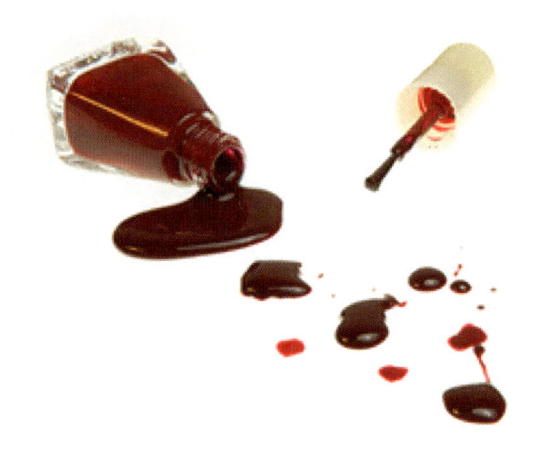

PEG
Compounds

The Cosmetic Chemicals Guide

PEG Compounds

Used As: Used as thickeners, solvents, softeners and moisture-carriers.

Dangers:
- ➡ Skin irritant
- ➡ Absorption enhancer
- ➡ Contaminated with 1,4 Dioxane

Found In:
- ☑ Hand sanitizer
- ☑ Lotions, creams
- ☑ Facial washes
- ☑ Body oils and lubricants
- ☑ Tooth gels and toothpastes
- ☑ Deodorant
- ☑ Hair care

Also known as:

Any ingredients with the prefix "PEG" followed by a number (e.g.. 7, 150, 8.)

Related chemical:

Propylene Glycol

Did You Know? PEG's are widely rumored to be numbing agents that desensitize the area, but there is no scientific data to back this up. They do increase absorption of other ingredients though and are likely to be contaminated with cancer-causing chemicals during their manufacturing process.

PEG Compounds

Hazards

Increase skin absorption	PEG compounds easily penetrate the skin and allow other chemicals to also penetrate quicker. PEG's should not be used on broken skin.
Cancer concerns	Possible contaminants such as *1,4 Dioxane* or *Ethylene Oxide* are known human carcinogens.
Allergies and skin irritation	Animal studies show skin irritation at low doses.
Organ development	Both reproductive and non-reproductive toxicity is indicated in animal studies.

Environment Canada Domestic Substances List:	*Flagged by CEPA for further investigation.*

PEG Compounds

So what have you learned about PEG Compounds?

➡ PEG's are petroleum-based compounds used as thickeners, moisture-carriers, solvents and softeners.

➡ There are many variations to PEG compounds, identified by the prefix "PEG" and followed by a number (e.g.. 6, 80, 150).

➡ PEG's are not safe when used on damaged or broken skin.

➡ PEG compounds easily penetrate the skin and aid other chemical ingredients to penetrate easier as well.

➡ Depending on the manufacturing process, PEGs can be contaminated with known human carcinogens.

➡ There is no evidence to support the rumor that PEGs are numbing agents and used to numb babies eyes in "No Tears" shampoo formulas. However, contamination concerns of *ethylene oxide*, a known human carcinogen, raises some questions.

➡ PEGs have shown to have developmental toxicity both to the reproductive and non-reproductive organs.

The Cosmetic Chemicals Guide

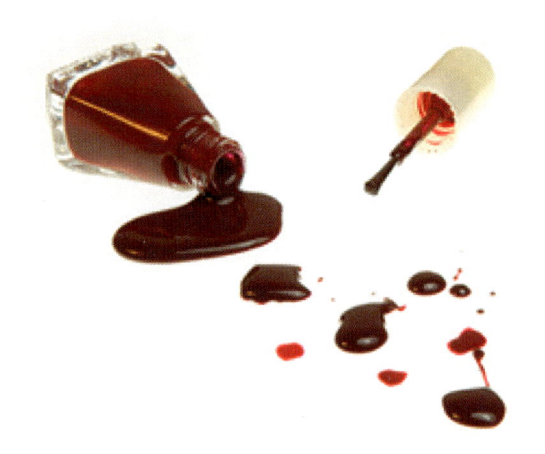

Petrolatum

The Cosmetic Chemicals Guide

Petrolatum

Used As: Barrier to lock in moisture, makes hair shiny, absorbs UV rays.

Dangers: ➡ Can be contaminated with polycyclic aromatic hydrocarbons (PAHs).

PAHs:

➡ Cause allergic reactions
➡ Cause skin irritation
➡ Are carcinogenic

Found In:
- ☑ Hair gels
- ☑ Lip gloss and shimmers
- ☑ Moisturizers, lotions and creams
- ☑ Baby ointment
- ☑ Hair gels and lotions

Also known as:

Mineral Jelly,

Petrolatum

Amber,

Petrolatum White,

Petroleum Jelly,

Yellow Petrolatum,

Mineral Grease

(Petrolatum)

Did You Know? The European Union only allows use of petrolatum in cosmetics if the full refining history is known; to guarantee it is free of carcinogens.

Petrolatum

Hazards

On it's own, Petrolatum is not harmful, but it is likely to be contaminated with PAHs, which are a serious health concern and have been found to be unsafe for use in cosmetics.

Skin irritation & allergies	Can cause skin irritations and allergic reactions.
Environmental concerns	Toxic to aquatic organisms. Also persistent and bioaccumulative.
Cancer concerns	Defined as possible human carcinogen and strong evidence of cancer.
Endocrine disruption	Evidence to show hormonal disruption.
Organ toxicity	Can be toxic and have detrimental effect on non-reproductive organs.

Environment Canada Domestic Substances List: *Flagged by CEPA for further review.*

Petrolatum

So what have you learned about Petrolatum?

➡ Petrolatum by itself is not a concern, but the likelihood of it being contaminated with PAHs is a large health concern.

➡ The European Union only allows petrolatum to be used in cosmetics if the full refining history is known; to ensure no contaminants are present in the product.

➡ This ingredient is being further reviewed by the CEPA, though no restrictions are set on use of this product in Canada or the USA.

➡ Mineral oil and petroleum distillates are related petroleum by-products and may also be contaminated with PAHs.

➡ Unless the full refining history is known, there is no way to be sure that the petrolatum used in cosmetics and personal care products does not contain dangerous by-products.

The Cosmetic Chemicals Guide

Siloxanes

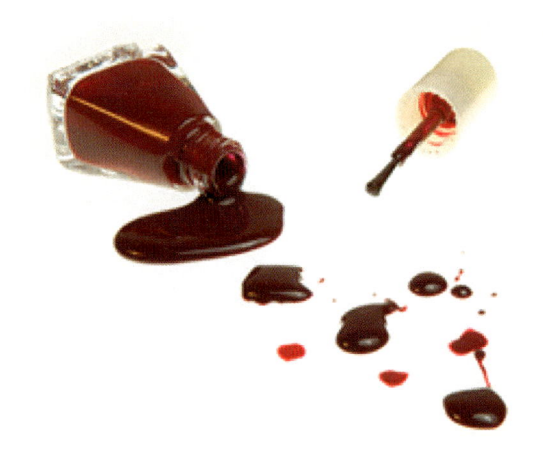

Siloxanes

Used As: Hair conditioner, skin conditioner. Makes hair products dry quicker and deodorants roll on easier.

Dangers:
- ➡ Harmful to the environment
- ➡ Toxic to organs
- ➡ Endocrine disruption
- ➡ Animal studies show tumor formation
- ➡ Neurotoxic
- ➡ Irritant to skin, eyes, lungs

Found In:
- ☑ Deodorants
- ☑ Facial and skin moisturizers
- ☑ Lip Plumpers
- ☑ Lubricants
- ☑ Hair care products
- ☑ Baby sunscreen lotions
- ☑ Cosmetics

Also known as:

Cyclopentasiloxane, Decamethyl-Decamethylcyclopentasiloxane, Decamethyl-Cyclopetasiloxane, Dimethylcyclopolysiloxane, Dow Corning 344 (345) Fluid, D4, D5, D6.

Related ingredients:

Polydimethylsiloxane (PDMS). *Dimethicone is a common PDMS used in cosmetics.

end in names "-siloxane" or "-cone".

Did You Know? Further studies need to be conducted to lessen the data gap surrounding siloxanes in personal care products. In 2009, D4 and D5 siloxanes were proposed to be moved to the List of Toxic Substances.

The Cosmetic Chemicals Guide

Siloxanes

Hazards

Environment	Suspected to be persistent and accumulative; toxic to wildlife.
Cancer concerns	Animal studies show tumor formation.
Skin irritation	Animal studies show skin irritation.
Endocrine disruption	Animal studies show endocrine disruption.
Neurotoxicity	Animal studies displayed neurological effects.

Environment Canada Domestic Substances List: *Flagged for further attention by the CEPA.*

Siloxanes

So what have you learned about Siloxanes?

→ Siloxanes are silicone-based compounds and used in many cosmetics and personal care items to smooth, soften and moisten.

→ Hair products, deodorants, moisturizers and facial treatments often contain siloxanes.

→ Recognize siloxane related chemicals by names ending in "*-siloxane*" or "*-cone*."

→ There is a large data gap of the effects of siloxane on humans, but animal studies have shown toxic effects on reproductive organs, skin irritations, organs, cellular changes and tumor formation.

→ Siloxanes are currently flagged for further attention by the CEPA.

→ *Dimethicone* is a very popular ingredient in cosmetics, it is related to the siloxane family.

The Cosmetic Chemicals Guide

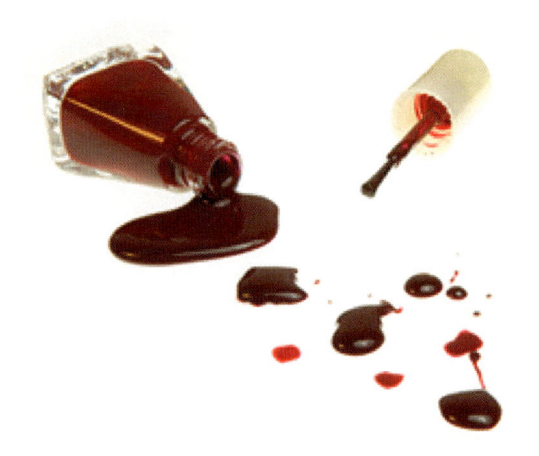

Sodium Lauryl Sulfate (SLS)

The Cosmetic Chemicals Guide

Sodium Lauryl Sulfate

Used As: Cleansing Agent. Helps products to strip away oils and make products foam.

Dangers:
- Skin and eye irritant
- Reproductive effects
- Endocrine disruption
- Environmental toxin
- Mammalian cells showed positive mutation results

Found In:
- ☑ Body washes and soaps
- ☑ Detergents
- ☑ Toothpastes
- ☑ Shampoos
- ☑ Dish soaps
- ☑ Food sources

Also known as:

SLS, Sodium Dodecyl Sulfate, Sulfuric Acid, Monodecyl Ester, Sodium Salt; Sodium Salt Sulfuric Acid, Monododecyl Ester Sodium Salt Sulfuric Acid, Sodium Lauryl Sulfate Sodium, A13-00356, Sodium Laureth Sulfate (SLES).

Did You Know? SLS can also be contaminated with carcinogens like 1,4 dioxane during the manufacturing process?

77

The Cosmetic Chemicals Guide

Sodium Lauryl Sulfate

Hazards

Allergic sensitivity reactions	Causes redness on skin, may cause respiratory irritation if inhaled.
Dry skin & eczema dermatitis	SLS is irritating and drying to the skin. Prolonged used may cause dermatitis.
Eye irritation	Causes redness in eyes and pain when it comes in contact with the eyes.
Environmental concerns	Toxic when comes in contact with aquatic organisms. The National Institute for Occupational Safety and Health recommends that it not be allowed to enter the environment.
Cancer concerns	If contaminated with 1,4 Dioxane, can cause cancer.

Environment Canada Domestic Substances List: *Classified as expected to be toxic or harmful*

Sodium Lauryl Sulfate

So what have you learned about SLS or SLES?

➡ Used to strip oils from surfaces; found in many soaps, washes, detergents and cleansers. Makes products bubble and foam as well.

➡ Causes skin irritation and eye irritation.

➡ May cause dermatitis if prolonged exposure occurs.

➡ Toxic to aquatic organisms; suspected to be an environmental toxin.

➡ Animal studies show endocrine disruption.

➡ Animal studies show reproductive effects.

➡ Flagged for further attention by the CEPA.

➡ May contain 1,4 Dioxane as a contaminant. 1,4 Dioxane is a known carcinogen.

The Cosmetic Chemicals Guide

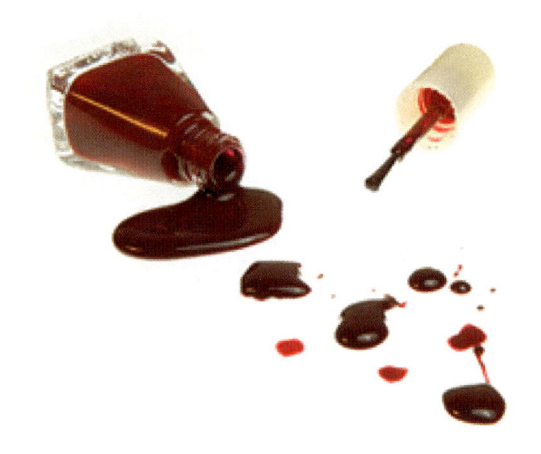

Triclosan

The Cosmetic Chemicals Guide

Triclosan

Used As: Preservative, anti-bacterial agent.

Dangers:
➡ Skin and eye irritant
➡ Toxic or harmful to organs
➡ Reproductive effects
➡ Endocrine disruption
➡ Toxic to wildlife

Found In:
- ☑ Face washes and cleansers
- ☑ Bath products
- ☑ Hair care products
- ☑ Deodorants, antiperspirants
- ☑ Soaps, washes
- ☑ Cosmetics
- ☑ Lotions, moisturizers
- ☑ Shaving cream

Also known as:

5-Chlor-2- (2,4- Dichlorophenoxy) Phenol, Phenol, 2,4,4'- Trichloro-2'- Hydroxy Diphenyl Ether, 5 Chloro2 (2,4 Dichlorophenoxy), CH 3565.

Did You Know? Triclosan is used in many products and does not easily degrade, allowing small quantities to build up and quite likely exceed the "allowable and safe" levels determined by the government.

The Cosmetic Chemicals Guide

Triclosan

Hazards

Organ toxicity	Expected to be toxic/harmful to organs and reproductive organs.
Endocrine disruption	Endocrine disruption indicated in studies.
Irritant	Classified as an irritant.
Cancer concerns	In vitro tests show non-mammalian cells mutated.
Environment	Toxic to the environment.

Environment Canada Domestic Substances List: *Flagged for further attention by the CEPA.*

Triclosan

So what have you learned about Triclosan?

➡ Triclosan is used in many cosmetics and personal care products, and while the current safe level is 0.3 percent, it has the ability to build up in the body and exceed those levels.

➡ Use is restricted in Canadian cosmetics, though some products, like anti-bacterial hand sanitizer, don't classify as "cosmetics" and this restriction may not apply to them.

➡ Triclosan was one of the chemical ingredients found in blood or urine in the "Teenage Chemical Test" done by the Environmental Working Group.

➡ Triclosan has been flagged by the CEPA for further attention.

➡ Triclosan can be present as an impurity in grapefruit seed extract.

Finding More Information

Thankfully, consumer awareness is on the rise and finding safer alternatives grows easier each day. While most manufacturers have not yet reformulated their products, many companies are starting up that offer "chemical-free" products.

Likewise, many natural health products store are offering a wide selection of products for the whole family, which allows you to review the products and get most of them at one convenient location.

Online Stores

As a mother of two children, I faced this battle a few years back and have been searching ever since for safe products. It was this search that resulted in Natural e GREEN, my online store offering safe product alternatives. Like mine, other stores exist online that also offer a great selection of safe alternative products. However, when shopping at stores like these, remember: they may carry a only a few brands that truly are chemical-free. So get familiar with the ingredients and do your research until you find brands you are familiar with and find stores you can trust!

EWG's Cosmetics Database

One of the first places I visited was the Environmental Working Group's Cosmetic Database. This vast collection of evaluated test the products you are using today and see how they rank for toxicity.

Finding More Information

The EWG's database ranks products and chemicals from 0-10 (0 being lowest, 10 being very toxic!) They also perform many studies and tests and publish their reports and findings.

You can visit the EWG's site @ http://www.cosmeticsdatabase.com

David Suzuki

This report went viral across the Internet when it was first published and is still a great reference. The "Dirty Dozen" is a report compiled by David Suzuki - you can view it here:
http://www.davidsuzuki.org/issues/health/science/toxics/dirty-dozen-cosmetic-chemicals/

Campaign for Safe Cosmetics

Join the movement for safe cosmetics and follow this group. Plus, see what companies have signed the Compact for Safe Cosmetics and which have not.

Visit them here:
http://www.safecosmetics.org/article.php?list=type&type=32

Conclusion

Although this is the end of this book, it is not the end of the challenge we face every day. Hopefully, this book has helped you to understand the product labels a little better and will make purchasing products a little easier.

Our generation today is the start of something big, the beginning of consumers telling manufacturers what they want. While only a few manufacturers have complied so far, most realize they too will eventually have to follow.

With consumer knowledge and pressure on both government and individual companies, there is hope that one day you will be able to walk into a store, pick up a product, and not have to worry that it contains unknown and harmful chemicals.

Our bodies are designed to filter out toxins and keep our organs and life system functioning well. However, the body can only work so hard and filter out so much before it becomes an impossible battle. The same is especially true for children and anyone who has pre-existing health conditions. Their bodies will have a harder time eliminating the toxins and keeping their system running smooth.

By reading this book, you have just taken your first step on the journey to better health. Maybe you picked up this book out of curiosity, maybe you got it as a gift; Whatever the reason, you now have more information that you did before and knowledge is power. Share what you have learned and strive to teach the younger generation so they can make safer choices when they grow up and hopefully, one day, live in a world without the harmful chemicals that we live with today.

Resources

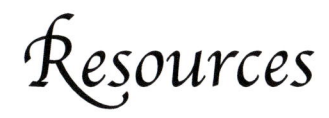

EWG: Cosmetic Database http://www.ewg.org/

EWG: Body Burden - The Pollution in Newborns
http://www.ewg.org/reports/bodyburden2/execsumm.php

David Suzuki: 'Dirty Dozen" cosmetic chemicals to avoid
http://www.davidsuzuki.org/issues/health/science/toxics/dirty-dozen-cosmetic-chemicals/

EWG: Teen Girls' Body Burden of Hormone-Altering Cosmetics Chemicals
http://www.ewg.org/reports/teens

Betton, C., "7th Amendment to the EU Cosmetics Directive," Cosmetic Science Technology (2005): 234-36.

Environmental Working Group. Report. "Pollution in People"
http://www.ewg.org/files/2009-Minority-Cord-Blood-Report.pdf

U.S Food and Drug Administration: Parabens
http://www.fda.gov/cosmetics/productandingredientsafety/selectedcosmeticingredients/ucm128042.htm

PHEND Pharmaceuticals: Dangers of PEG Compounds in Cosmetics Women at Increased Breast Cancer Risk?
http://www.phend.co.za/health/Chemical5.htm

Material Safety Data Sheets (MSDS): Ethylene Oxide
http://hazard.com/msds/mf/cards/file/0155.html

U.S Food and Drug Administration: FDA Authority Over Cosmetics
http://www.fda.gov/Cosmetics/GuidanceComplianceRegulatoryInformation/ucm074162.htm

Mayo Clinic: Lead in Lipstick

http://www.mayoclinic.com/health/lead-in-lipstick/AN01618

Campaign for Safe Cosmetics: Toxic Tub: Product Test Results
http://safecosmetics.org/article.php?id=426

ABC Good Morning America: Brazilian Blowout Hair-Straitening Product Under Fire
http://abcnews.go.com/GMA/Consumer/brazilian-blowout-hair-straightening-samples-formaldehyde/story?id=11771569

Health Canada: Brazilian Blowout Solution Contains Formaldehyde
http://www.hc-sc.gc.ca/ahc-asc/media/advisories-avis/_2010/2010_167-eng.php

CBC News: Rival follows suit in Brazilian Blowout recall
http://www.cbc.ca/canada/calgary/story/2010/10/13/calgary-brazilian-blowout-keratin-warning-shipments-halted.html

Time: Parabens Outlawed in Children's Products in Denmark
http://healthland.time.com/2010/12/22/parabens-outlawed-in-childrens-products-in-denmark/

BBC News: Concern over deodorant chemicals
http://news.bbc.co.uk/2/hi/health/3383393.stm

Environmental Health Perspectives: Urinary Concentrations of Four Parabens in the U.S Population: NHANES 2005-2006
http://ehp03.niehs.nih.gov/article/fetchArticle.action?articleURI=info%3Adoi%2F10.1289%2Fehp.0901560

Natural News: Procter and Gamble to reduce 1,4 dioxane levels in Herbal Essences shampoos
http://www.naturalnews.com/028560_Herbal_Essences_shampoo.html

Canada.com: Chemical found in baby shampoos not toxic: Health Canada
http://www.canada.com/health/Chemical+found+baby+shampoos+toxic+Health+Canada/1963940/story.html

The Alliance For a Healthy Tomorrow: Cancer-causing 1,4 Dioxane Found in Children's Bath Products
http://www.healthytomorrow.org/2007/02/bath_products.html

Toronto Sun: Be wary of scents at holiday parties
http://www.torontosun.com/life/greenplanet/2010/12/09/16487506.html

Pure Zing: List of the More Widely Dangerous Ingredients in Body & Food Products
http://www.purezing.com/living/toxins/living_toxins_dangerousingredients.html

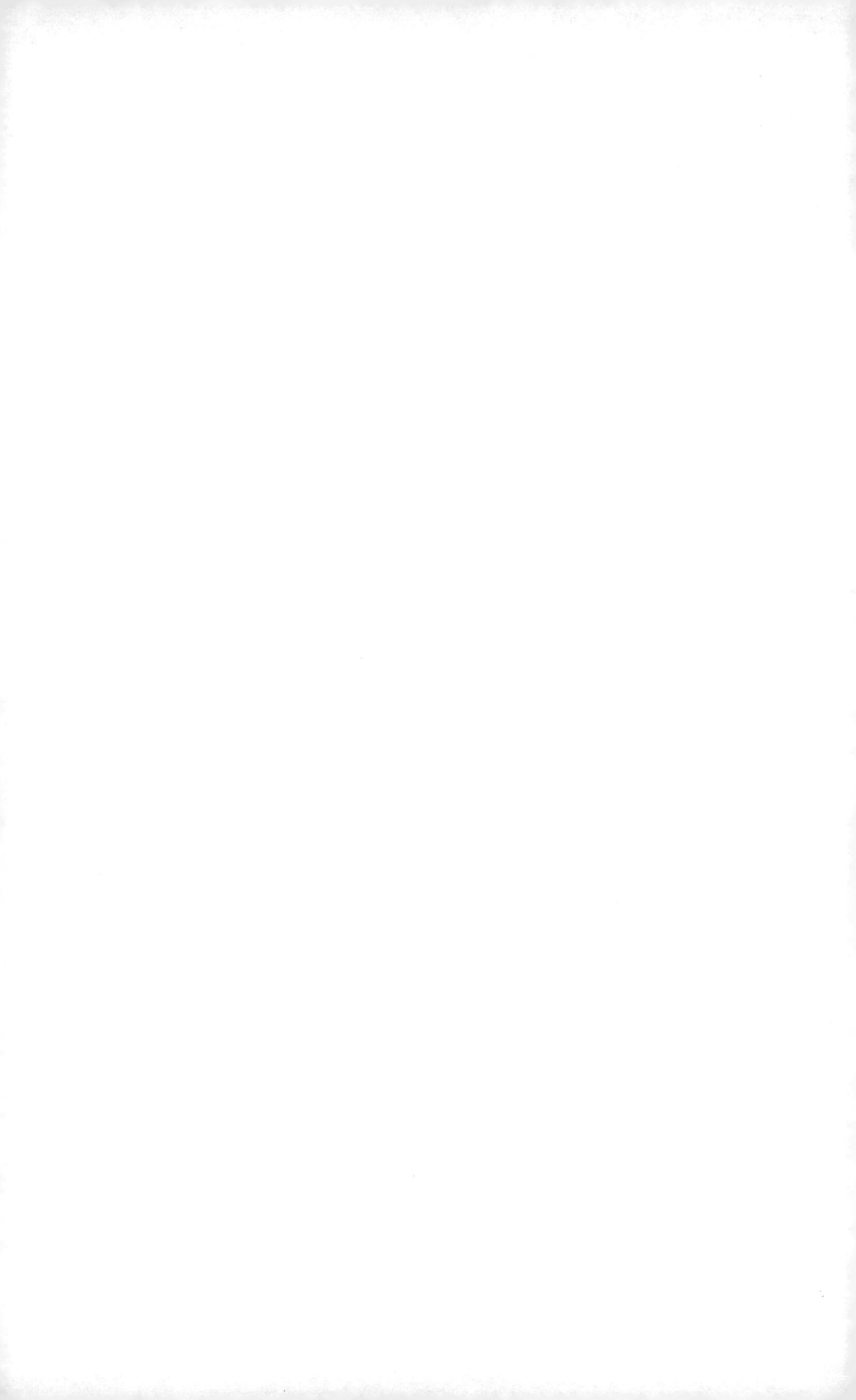

Made in the USA
Charleston, SC
24 January 2011